It's easy to get lost in the cancer world

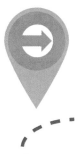

Let NCCN Guidelines for Patients® be your guide

✓ Step-by-step guides to the cancer care options likely to have the best results

✓ Based on treatment guidelines used by health care providers worldwide

✓ Designed to help you discuss cancer treatment with your doctors

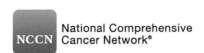

NCCN Guidelines for Patients® are developed by the National Comprehensive Cancer Network® (NCCN®)

NCCN

✓ An alliance of leading cancer centers across the United States devoted to patient care, research, and education

Cancer centers that are part of NCCN:
NCCN.org/cancercenters

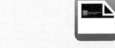

NCCN Clinical Practice Guidelines in Oncology (NCCN Guidelines®)

✓ Developed by doctors from NCCN cancer centers using the latest research and years of experience

✓ For providers of cancer care all over the world

✓ Expert recommendations for cancer screening, diagnosis, and treatment

Free online at
NCCN.org/guidelines

NCCN Guidelines for Patients

✓ Present information from the NCCN Guidelines in an easy-to-learn format

✓ For people with cancer and those who support them

✓ Explain the cancer care options likely to have the best results

Free online at
NCCN.org/patientguidelines

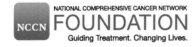

and supported by funding from NCCN Foundation®

These NCCN Guidelines for Patients are based on the NCCN Guidelines® for B-Cell Lymphomas Version 4.2020 (August 13, 2020).

NCCN Foundation seeks to support the millions of patients and their families affected by a cancer diagnosis by funding and distributing NCCN Guidelines for Patients. NCCN Foundation is also committed to advancing cancer treatment by funding the nation's promising doctors at the center of innovation in cancer research. For more details and the full library of patient and caregiver resources, visit NCCN.org/patients.

National Comprehensive Cancer Network (NCCN) / NCCN Foundation
3025 Chemical Road, Suite 100
Plymouth Meeting, PA 19462
215.690.0300

Endorsed by

The Leukemia & Lymphoma Society
The Leukemia & Lymphoma Society (LLS) is dedicated to developing better outcomes for blood cancer patients and their families through research, education, support and advocacy and is happy to have this comprehensive resource available to patients. lls.org/informationspecialists

To make a gift or learn more, please visit NCCNFoundation.org/donate or e-mail PatientGuidelines@nccn.org.

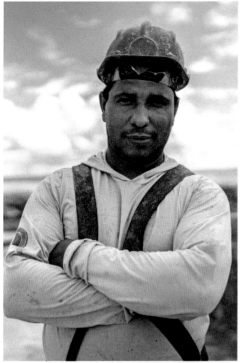
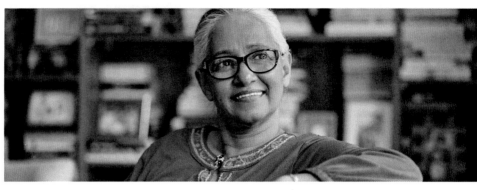
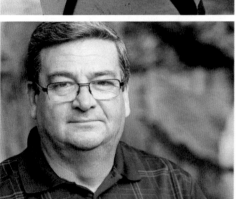

Lymphoma
non-Hodgkin
Hodgkin
common
blood
enlarged
diseases
lymphomas
Treatment
World
tumors
virus
cancer
Diagnosis
developed
survival
therapy
categories
factors
amount
cells

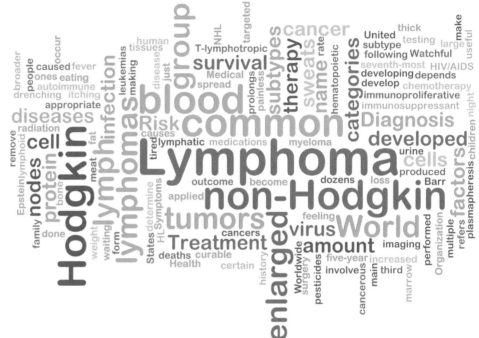
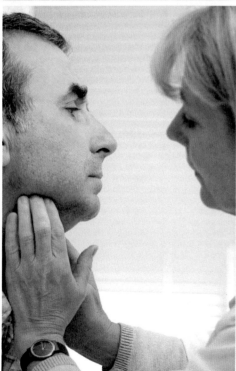
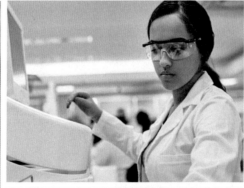
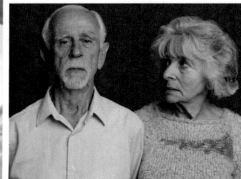
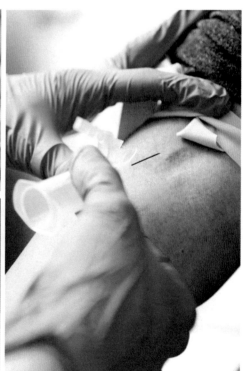

Contents

1
DLBCL basics

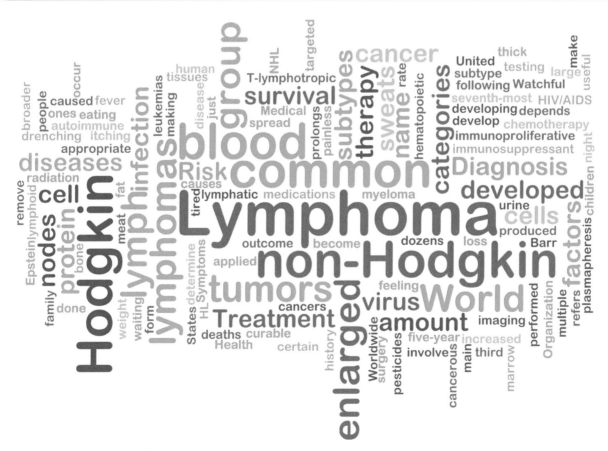

Diffuse large B-cell lymphoma (DLBCL) is a type of cancer called non-Hodgkin lymphoma. It is a fast-growing cancer, but with the right treatment, it can be well controlled.

The lymph system

Lymphoma is a cancer of the lymph (or lymphatic) system. The lymph system is a network of fluid and tissues in your body. It supports the cardiovascular system by transporting fluids to the bloodstream. It is also a major part of your body's disease-fighting (immune) system.

Lymph and lymph vessels

Lymph is a fluid within a "super highway" of ducts throughout the body. These ducts are called lymph (or lymphatic) vessels. Lymph vessels carry lymph away from body tissue and release it into the bloodstream.

Lymph is formed from tissue (or interstitial) fluid. Tissue fluid fills the spaces between cells in body tissue. It is made from the part of the blood called plasma. When tissue fluid increases, some of it drains into lymph vessels and becomes lymph.

There is fatty lymph called chyle. After you eat, your stomach turns food into a liquid. Then, the liquid moves into your small intestine. Within your small intestine, fat and some vitamins drain into lymph vessels and form chyle, Chyle travels in lymph vessels to the bloodstream.

Lymph tissue

Lymph tissue has high numbers of white blood cells called lymphocytes. There are small clumps of lymph tissue in your gut, thyroid, breasts, lungs, eyes, and skin. You also have larger masses of lymph tissue in the:

> Spleen

> Tonsils

> Thymus

> Lymph nodes

As lymph travels through lymph vessels, it passes through hundreds of structures called lymph nodes. Lymph nodes filter out germs from lymph. Some areas of the body have more lymph nodes than others. The highest numbers of lymph nodes are found in the:

> Neck (cervical lymph nodes)

> Groin (inguinal lymph nodes)

> Armpits (axillary lymph nodes)

Types of lymphoma

Lymphoma forms from cells called lymphocytes. They are part of the immune system and help to fight disease. The three types of lymphocytes are B cells, T cells, and natural killer cells.

There are two main types of lymphomas:

> Hodgkin lymphoma

> Non-Hodgkin lymphoma

Doctors can tell the type of lymphoma by looking at the cancer cells under a microscope.

Hodgkin lymphoma is a cancer of B cells called Reed-Sternberg cells. These cells are very large. Unlike a normal cell, they may have an "owl-eye" look from having two nuclei.

Non-Hodgkin lymphoma is the more common type. It is a group of more than 90 cancers. These cancers do not have Reed-Sternberg cells. They are cancers of B cells, T cells, or natural killer cells.

Diffuse large B-cell lymphoma

Diffuse large B-cell lymphoma (DLBCL) is a non-Hodgkin lymphoma. It is a cancer of B cells. B cells transform through many stages to become cells that are able to fight disease. DLBCL is a cancer of mature B cells from the lymph system. Read **Part 2** to learn about the tests of cells that are used to confirm (diagnose) DLBCL.

DLBCL is named for how it looks under a microsope. It has a wide (diffuse) pattern of growth. The cancer cells grow throughout tissue rather than in clusters. It is also named after the large size of the cancer cells.

DLBCL is a fast-growing cancer. The cancer cells often build up in lymph tissue. Lymph nodes with cancer may become so large that they can be easily felt. The cancer cells often grow fast compared to other lymphomas. The cancer cells can involve body parts outside the lymph system.

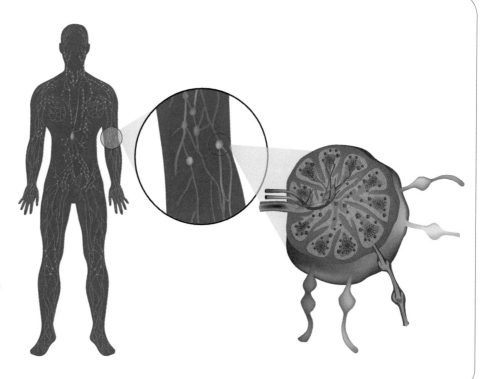

Lymphoma

Lymphoma is a cancer of the lymph (or lymphatic) system. This system transports a fluid called lymph to the bloodstream. It also helps the immune system fight disease. Lymph vessels and nodes are depicted in green in the picture.

Subtypes of DLBCL

There are many subtypes of DLBCL. The treatment options in this book apply to these types:

> *ALK*-positive DLBCL

> DLBCL with follicular lymphoma

> DLBCL with gastric MALT lymphoma

> DLBCL with nongastric MALT lymphoma

> DLBCL, not otherwise specified (NOS)

> DLBCL associated with chronic inflammation

> DLBCL with *IRF4/MUM1* rearrangement

> EBV-positive DLBCL, NOS

> Intravascular large B-cell lymphoma

> T-cell-/histiocyte-rich large B-cell lymphoma

Treatment options in this book may also apply to follicular lymphoma grade 3. Grade 3 is the highest grade. It is divided into grade 3A and grade 3B.

This book does not include information on:

> DLBCL arising from chronic lymphocytic leukemia (Richter's transformation)

> Grey zone lymphoma

> High-grade B-cell lymphoma with translocations of *MYC* and either or both *BCL2* and *BCL6*

> HIV-positive DLBCL

> Primary cutaneous DLBCL, leg type

> Primary cutaneous marginal zone lymphoma (PCMZL)

> Primary cutaneous follicle center lymphoma (PCFCL)

> Primary DLBCL of the central nervous system

> Primary mediastinal large B-cell lymphoma (PMBL)

Types of treatment

This section briefly describes treatments for DLBCL. Not everyone receives the same treatment. Your doctor will tailor treatment to you based on tests in **Part 2** and **Part 3**. Treatment options based on the extent of cancer and other factors are listed in **Part 4**.

Clinical trial
One treatment choice may be a clinical trial. Joining a clinical trial is strongly supported by NCCN. NCCN believes that you will receive the best management if treated in a clinical trial.

A clinical trial is a type of research that studies a promising test or treatment in people. It gives people access to health care that otherwise couldn't usually be received. Ask your treatment team if there is an open clinical trial that you can join.

Antibody treatment
Antibodies are proteins of the immune system. They help your body fight germs and other threats. Monoclonal antibodies can be made in a lab to treat certain types of cancer.

There are two antibody treatments for DLBCL.

- Rituximab
- Tafasitamab-cxix

Rituximab attaches to a surface protein on cells called CD20, and tafasitamab-cxix attaches to CD19. They mark the cells so that your immune system can find and destroy them. They may directly kill cells, too.

Antibody-drug conjugates
Antibody-drug conjugates attach to surface proteins on cells then release a drug that causes cell death. There are two antibody-drug conjugates for DLBCL.

- Brentuximab vedotin
- Polatuzumab vedotin

Brentuximab vedotin attaches to a surface protein called CD30, and polatuzumab vedotin attaches to CD79b. Not all people with DLBCL have CD30 on the cancer cells.

Chemotherapy
Chemotherapy works by damaging and killing cancer cells. It can also cause cells to destroy themselves. Chemotherapy is often used with rituximab to treat DLBCL. This combined treatment is called chemoimmunotherapy.

There are many types of chemotherapy used to treat DLBCL. Drugs from more than one class of chemotherapy are used for treatment.

- Alkylating agents include bendamustine, carboplatin, cisplatin, cyclophosphamide, ifosfamide, oxaliplatin, and procarbazine.
- Anthracyclines include doxorubicin.

- Antimetabolites include gemcitabine, methotrexate, and cytarabine.
- Plant alkaloids include vincristine and etoposide.

Corticosteroids
Corticosteroids are a class of drugs that are often used to relieve inflammation. They also are toxic to lymphoma cells. Prednisone, methylprednisolone, and dexamethasone are corticosteroids used for treatment. They are part of some chemoimmunotherapy regimens.

Immunomodulators
Immunomodulators are drugs that modify some parts of the immune system. Lenalidomide is an immunomodulator that is sometimes used to treat or prevent a return of DLBCL. Lenalidomide may be given with rituximab or tafasitamab-cxix for treatment.

Targeted therapy
Targeted therapy is a class of drugs. It impedes the growth process that is specific to cancer cells. It harms normal cells less than chemotherapy.

Kinase inhibitors
Within cells, kinases are part of many chemical pathways, some of which control cell growth. They change the action of proteins by attaching phosphates to them. Kinase inhibitors are drugs that stop kinases within cancer cells. Ibrutinib is a drug that stops a kinase called Bruton's tyrosine kinase. This lowers the number of new cancer cells being made.

Small molecule inhibitor
Exportin 1 is a protein that helps to deliver messages from the cell nucleus. The messages

tell the cell to multiply or not die. Selinexor is a drug that targets exportin 1 and stops the messages from being sent.

Radiation therapy

Radiation therapy uses high-energy x-rays to treat DLBCL. The x-rays damage DNA in cancer cells. This either kills the cancer cells or stops new cancer cells from being made.

Involved-site radiation therapy (ISRT) treats lymphoma in the areas it was found at diagnosis. It may be received after chemoimmunotherapy or a blood stem cell transplant.

Blood stem cell transplant

Blood stem (or hematopoietic) cell transplants replace damaged or destroyed stem cells with healthy stem cells. The healthy stem cells form new bone marrow and blood cells. There are two types of transplants.

> Autologous transplant

> Allogeneic transplant

An autologous transplant is also called high-dose therapy with autologous stem cell rescue (HDT/ASCR). First, some of your healthy stem cells will be removed. You will then receive chemotherapy to kill the cancer cells. It will also kill the blood-producing cells in the bone marrow. Your healthy stem cells will then be returned to "rescue" your bone marrow.

An allogeneic transplant uses healthy stem cells from a donor. You'll first receive treatment called conditioning to kill your bone marrow cells. Next, you'll receive the donor cells. These cells will form new, healthy bone marrow.

They will also attack cancer cells that weren't killed by prior treatment.

Anti-CD19 CAR T-cell therapy

Treatment is made from your own T cells. Some of your T cells will be removed from your body, and chimeric antigen receptor (CAR) will be added to them in a lab. This programs the T cells to find lymphoma cells. The CAR T cells will be infused back into your body to find and kill cancer cells. The anti-CD19 CAR T-cell therapies are tisagenlecleucel and axicabtagene ciloleucel.

Review

> Lymphoma is a cancer of the lymph system. This system is a network of lymph, lymph vessels, and lymph tissues. It transports fluids to the bloodstream and helps kill germs in the body.

> Lymphoma forms from cells called lymphocytes. Lymphocytes are a type of white blood cell that help fight disease. The three types of lymphocytes are B cells, T cells, and natural killer cells.

> DLBCL is a type of non-Hodgkin lymphoma. It is a cancer of mature B cells. It is a fast-growing cancer that often involves lymph nodes. It can also involve body parts outside the lymph system.

> There are many subtypes of DLBCL. Follicular lymphoma grade 3 is often treated like DLBCL.

> Chemoimmunotherapy is a common treatment for DLBCL. But, not everyone receives the same treatment. Your doctors will tailor treatment to you.

2
Tests for DLBCL

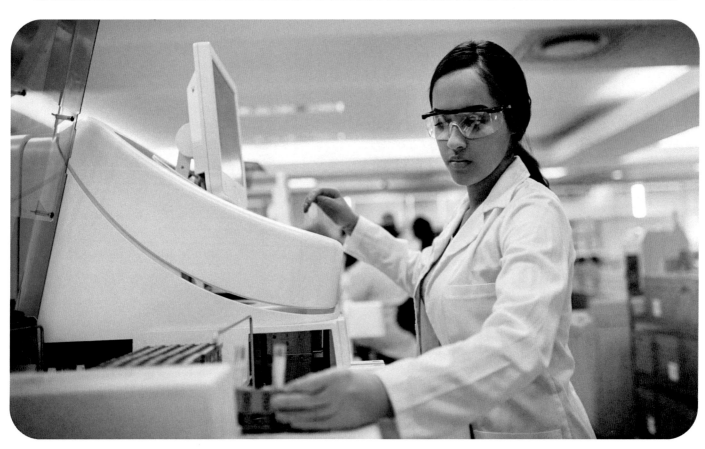

There are many types of lymphoma. Knowing which type you have is very important so you get the right treatment. This chapter describes the tests for DLBCL.

Lymphoma can arise in almost any part of the body. For that reason, it can cause different signs and symptoms among people. Signs and symptoms caused by lymphoma can also be caused by other diseases, too.

One of the first signs of lymphoma may be a swelling of lymph tissue. Lymph nodes may be so large that they can be easily felt or seen under the skin. Lymphoma can also cause abnormal blood counts.

If your doctor suspects that you have lymphoma, testing is needed. The procedures and tests that are needed to confirm (diagnose) DLBCL are listed in Guide 1.

Biopsy

A biopsy is a procedure that removes samples of fluid or tissue for testing. It's the only way to know if you have cancer.

Type of biopsy

The best way to diagnose lymphoma is to have an incisional or excisional biopsy. These biopsies remove tissue through a cut into your skin.

- An incisional biopsy removes only part of the tissue that may have cancer.

- An excisional biopsy removes all of the tissue, such as an entire lymph node.

There are other types of biopsies that remove very small samples with a needle. Fine-needle aspiration (FNA) removes a small group of cells. A core needle biopsy removes a solid tissue sample.

Needle biopsies are not the best method for diagnosing lymphoma. You may have cancer even if no cancer is found in these biopsy samples. In certain cases, a core needle biopsy may be used to obtain samples. For hard-to-reach lymph nodes, FNA and core needle biopsies may be used to obtain samples.

Guide 1 Tests for DLBCL
Excisional or incisional biopsy; for certain people, multiple core and FNA biopsies
IHC panel with or without flow cytometry to identify type of lymphoma
Karyotype or FISH for *MYC* rearrangement
Karyotype or FISH for *BCL2* and *BCL6* rearrangements if there is an *MYC* rearrangement
IHC panel to identify lymphoma subtype if needed

Lab tests

Blood and tissue samples will be sent to a doctor called a hematopathologist. Hematopathologists are experts at diagnosing cancers of blood and immune cells. They spend much of their time working with samples of blood, bone marrow, and lymph tissue.

The biopsy tissue will be tested to diagnose DLBCL. The hematopathologist will examine the tissue using a microscope to see if there are cancer cells. Cancer cells will be studied to learn if cancer started in lymph tissue or elsewhere. Lymphoma cells will be tested for certain proteins and genes, which are described next.

Lab results used for diagnosis are included in a pathology report. This report will be sent to your cancer doctor. Ask for a copy. It is used to plan your treatment. Your doctor will review the results with you. Take notes and ask questions.

Immunophenotyping

The hematopathologist will identify the proteins on the surface and inside of cancer cells. This is called immunophenotyping. It is done to assess the:

> type of lymphoma; and

> the normal cell from which the cancer formed (cell of origin).

The outlook and treatment of DLBCL may differ based on the cell of origin. Some DLBCLs start from B cells that are within the "factories" of lymph tissue. These factories are called germinal centers. Proteins tests reveal whether

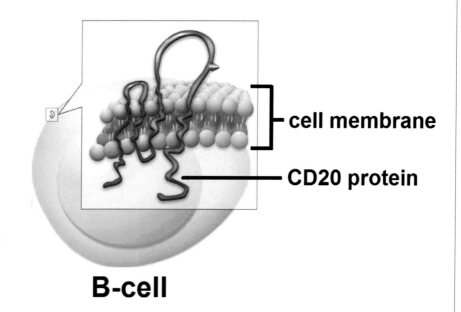

Immunophenotyping

Diffuse large B-cell lymphoma has common patterns of proteins on its cells. Immunophenotyping is the process of identifying the proteins.

Derivative work of NIAID - Rituxima Binding to CD20 on a B Cell Surface, CC BY 2.0, https://commons.wikimedia.org/w/index.php?curid=39933221

cell membrane

CD20 protein

B-cell

DLBCL formed from germinal center B cells (GCB) or non-GCBs.

The lab test that is often used to identify proteins is called immunohistochemistry (IHC). It is performed using tissue samples. Another lab test called flow cytometry may be done, too. A blood or tissue sample may be used for this test.

DLBCL has common patterns or a "signature" of proteins. For example, DLBCL often has proteins called CD20 and CD45 and does not have CD3. GCBs have CD10 while non-GCBs do not.

Gene rearrangements

Inside of most cells are 46 long strands (or 23 pairs) of DNA (deoxyribonucleic acid). A gene is a small segment of DNA with complex instructions. A gene rearrangement is the fusion of parts from two genes that creates a new gene.

To plan treatment, testing for an *MYC* rearrangement is needed. Lab tests that detect gene rearrangements are a karyotype and fluorescence in situ hybridization (FISH). If an *MYC* rearrangement is found, testing for *BCL2* and *BCL6* rearrangements is needed, too.

Lymphoma that has an *MYC* rearrangement and either a *BCL2* or *BCL6* rearrangement is called a "double-hit" high-grade B-cell lymphoma. If cells have all 3 rearrangements, the cancer is a "triple-hit" high-grade B-cell lymphoma. These lymphomas are treated differently than DLBCL.

Immunophenotyping

Immunophenotyping is the study of cell proteins to identify the cell type. It is used to diagnose blood cancers and lymphomas.

The two lab tests used to find proteins are called immunohistochemistry (IHC) and flow cytometry. A diagnosis is made based on which proteins are seen and not seen with these tests.

When DLBCL is suspected, testing for the following proteins is needed to identify the type of lymphoma:

IHC panel

- BCL2, BCL6, CD3, CD5, CD10, CD20, CD45, IRF4/MUM1, Ki-67, and MYC

Flow cytometry

- CD45, CD3, CD5, CD10, CD19, CD20, and kappa and lambda light chain proteins

It is sometimes useful to identify the lymphoma subtype. The following proteins should be included in the panel.

IHC panel

- ALK, CD30, CD138, cyclin D1, EBER-ISH, HHV8, SOX11, and kappa and lambda light chains

Review

- An incisional or excisional biopsy is the best method for diagnosing lymphoma.

- Biopsy samples should be tested by a doctor called a hematopathologist.

- The hematopathologist will perform a number of tests that assess for cell type, cell proteins, and changes in genes.

My diagnosis was sudden, unexpected and life shattering. I am a non-smoker and runner, and had just completed a ½ marathon before diagnosis. My only symptom was a persistent cough. My tumor was 10 cm by 14 cm and causing fluid to back up in my heart and lungs.

– Angie

   Survivor, Age 52 at diagnosis

3
Before treatment starts

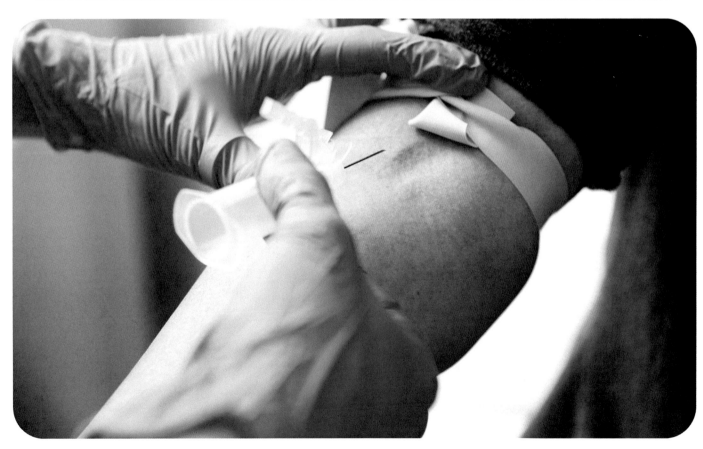

A specific group of tests is needed to plan treatment for DLBCL. This chapter describes the tests doctors use to learn more about the cancer and you. For younger people with cancer, the steps for having a healthy baby are discussed.

Health history and exam

It is important that your cancer doctors have all of your health information. A complete report of your health is called a medical history. A medical history and other health care that are used to plan and prepare for cancer treatment are listed in Guide 2.

Medical history

It is very common for doctors to ask about health problems and treatments. When you meet with your cancer doctors, be prepared to talk about:

> Illnesses

> Injuries

> Health conditions

> Symptoms

> Medications

DLBCL can cause "B symptoms." It is important that your doctor knows if you have them. The B symptoms are:

> Fevers

> Heavy sweats

> Unexplained weight loss

Lymphoma B symptoms

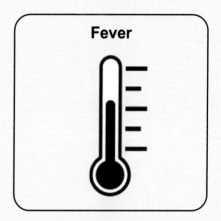

Fever

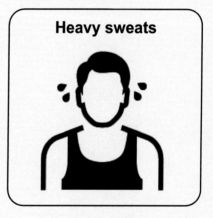

Heavy sweats

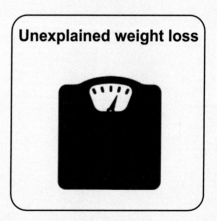

Unexplained weight loss

Guide 2
Health care before cancer treatment

Health history and exams	• Medical history including B symptoms • Physical exam including areas with many lymph nodes, liver, spleen • Performance status
Blood tests	• CDC with differential • Comprehensive metabolic panel • LDH • Uric acid • Beta-2 microglobulin if needed
Infectious disease tests	• Hepatitis B test • Hepatitis C test if needed • HIV test if needed
Imaging	• Whole-body PET/CT with or without diagnostic CT • CT or MRI scan of head or neck as needed
Heart test	• Echocardiogram or MUGA scan if certain chemotherapy is planned
Prognostic assessments	• Lugano Modification of Ann Arbor Staging System • International Prognostic Index (IPI) • Central nervous system (CNS) IPI
Biopsies	• Bone marrow biopsy with or without aspiration • Lumbar puncture as needed
Fertility and pregnancy care	• Pregnancy test if chemotherapy or radiation therapy is planned • Fertility counseling as needed

Some cancers and other health conditions can run in families. Be prepared to tell the health history of your close blood relatives. Such family includes your siblings, parents, and grandparents.

Physical exam

A physical exam of your body is done to look for signs of disease. It is also used to help assess what treatments may be options. During this exam, expect the following to be checked:

> Your body temperature

> Your blood pressure

> Your pulse and breathing rate

> Your weight

> How your lungs, heart, and gut sound

> How your eyes, skin, nose, ears, and mouth look

> The size of your organs

> Level of pain when you are touched

Lymphoma can cause lymph tissue and the liver to enlarge. Your doctor will gently press on the areas of your body that have lots of lymph nodes. High numbers of nodes are in the middle of your chest, neck, throat, armpit, groin, pelvis, and along your gut. Your doctor will also feel your spleen and liver to assess their size.

Performance status

Based on your history and exam, your doctor will rate your performance status. Performance status is your ability to do day-to-day activities.

Doctors use the performance status to assess if certain treatments are options. The Eastern Cooperative Oncology Group (ECOG)

Performance Status is a common scoring system. It consists of five scores.

> A score of 0 means you are fully active.

> A score of 1 means you are able to do all self-care activities but are unable to do hard physical work.

> A score of 2 means you are able to do all self-care activities and spend most of waking time out of bed but are unable to do any work.

> A score of 3 means you are unable to do all self-care activities and any work and spend most of waking time in bed.

> A score of 4 means you are fully disabled.

Blood tests

Blood tests are used to learn if cancer treatment might be needed now. They are also used to find diseases including those related to lymphoma. It's important to treat all illnesses.

Samples of blood are removed with a blood draw. A blood draw is performed with a needle inserted into a vein. You may need to fast from food and most liquids for hours before the draw.

Complete blood count with differential

A complete blood count (CBC) measures parts of the blood. Test results include counts of white blood cells, red blood cells, and platelets. Cancer and other health problems can cause low or high counts.

There are several types of white blood cells. A differential counts the number of each type of cell. It also checks if the counts are in balance with each other.

Comprehensive metabolic panel

Chemicals in your blood come from your liver, bone, kidneys, and other organs. A comprehensive metabolic panel often includes tests for up to 14 chemicals. The tests show if the level of chemicals is too low or high. Abnormal levels can be caused by cancer or other health problems.

LDH

Lactate dehydrogenase (LDH) is a protein that is in most cells. Dying cells release LDH into blood. High levels can be caused by cancer or other health problems. If related to lymphoma, high levels may be a sign that treatment may be needed now or soon.

Uric acid

Uric acid is a chemical that is found in foods and also made by the body. Too much uric acid in the blood is called hyperuricemia. You may have a high level of uric acid before starting treatment. Levels can be high due to a fast-growing cancer, kidney disease, or other health problems.

Your uric acid levels may also be checked during treatment. Some intense cancer treatments cause tumor lysis syndrome (TLS). TLS may cause kidney damage and severe blood electrolyte disturbances. TLS may be prevented by high amounts of fluids and medicines.

Beta-2 microglobulin

Beta-2 microglobulin is a small protein found on most cells. It is released by cells into the blood, especially by B cells. High levels can be caused by a fast-growing cancer or other health problems.

Infectious disease tests

An infectious disease is an illness caused by germs like viruses, bacteria, and fungi. Some types of cancer treatments can increase your chance of getting new infections. Chronic infections are a concern, too. Some can become active again after certain cancer treatments.

Hepatitis

Hepatitis B and hepatitis C can become active again while taking chemoimmunotherapy. These infections often need treatment even if they are causing no symptoms. Tell your treatment team if you have hepatitis. If you're unsure, testing is advised. A sample of your blood is needed for testing.

HIV

If you have HIV, treating it is an important part of treating DLBCL. HIV treatment will improve how well cancer treatment works. In addition, DLBCL may be managed differently. Tell your treatment team if you have HIV and about your treatment. If you are unsure, ask your treatment team if you should get tested.

Imaging

Imaging makes pictures of the insides of your body. It is used to detect cancer in deep tissue, lymph nodes, or distant body parts. Some imaging also reveals some features of a tumor and its cells.

A radiologist is a doctor who's an expert in reading images. This doctor will convey the test results to your other doctors.

Some imaging tests use contrast. It is a substance that is often injected into the bloodstream. It makes the images easier to read. Tell your doctor if you've had problems with contrast in the past. Also, allergies to shellfish may mean you'll be allergic to some types of contrast.

Whole-body PET/CT with or without diagnostic CT

Positron emission tomography (PET) and computed tomography (CT) are two types of imaging. When used together, they are called a PET/CT scan. Some cancer centers have one machine that does both tests.

PET requires injecting a radiotracer into your bloodstream. The radiotracer is detected with a special camera during the scan. PET can show even small amounts of cancer. The tracer is passed out of your body in your urine.

CT makes a more detailed image than a plain x-ray. It takes many pictures of your body from different angles using x-rays. A computer then combines the pictures to make a 3-D image.

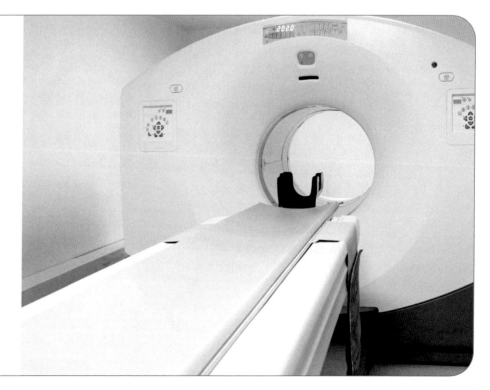

PET/CT

Pictures of the insides of your body can be made with imaging. During the scan, you will lie on a table that will move into the tunnel of the machine. The pictures will be viewed by a doctor who will look for signs of cancer.

The PET/CT scan will be used to image your whole body. Your doctor may also want you to get a diagnostic CT scan of your chest, abdomen, and pelvis. Contrast and a higher dose of radiation are used for a diagnostic CT. They help produce a more detailed image.

CT or MRI of neck or head

Imaging of the neck or head is helpful at times. It is used to look for cancer in lymph nodes. CT with contrast or magnetic resonance imaging (MRI) can be used. MRI makes 3-D images like CT. Unlike CT, images are made using a magnetic field and radio waves.

Heart test

Some types of chemotherapy can damage your heart. To plan treatment, your doctor may test how well your heart pumps blood. You may get an echocardiogram or multigated acquisition (MUGA) scan. An echocardiogram uses sound waves to make pictures of your heart. A MUGA scan makes pictures using an injected radiotracer and special camera.

Prognostic assessments

A prognosis is a prediction of the pattern and outcome of a disease. For treatment planning, your doctors will assess the cancer prognosis. The cancer stage and IPI score are the two methods used.

Cancer stage

The cancer stage describes the extent of cancer in the body. It is often based on blood tests, imaging, and biopsy results. The Lugano modification of the Ann Arbor Staging System is used for most lymphomas. This system has 4 main cancer stages:

> Stage 1

> Stage 2

> Stage 3

> Stage 4

DLBCL is stage 1 or 2 among less than half of people at diagnosis (about 40%). The extent of these cancers is limited. They involve lymph nodes or an organ on one side of the diaphragm.

Most often, DLBCL is stage 3 or 4 at diagnosis. The extent of these cancers is advanced. Stage 3 cancers are on both sides of the diaphragm. Stage 4 cancers have widely spread outside of the lymph system.

Examples of the cancer stages are on the next pages.

Stage 1

There is cancer in one group of lymph tissue on the same side of the diaphragm.

Reproduced with permission by Cancer Research UK / Wikimedia Commons.

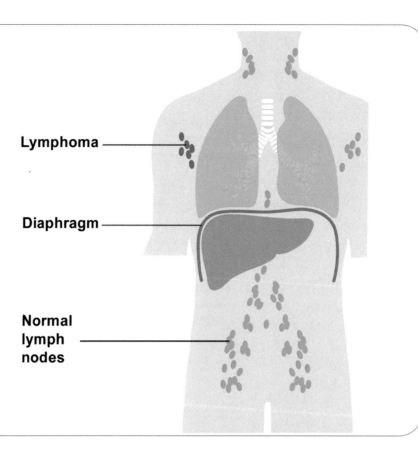

Lymphoma

Diaphragm

Normal lymph nodes

Stage 2

There is cancer in 2 or more groups of lymph tissue on the same side of the diaphragm.

Reproduced with permission by Cancer Research UK / Wikimedia Commons

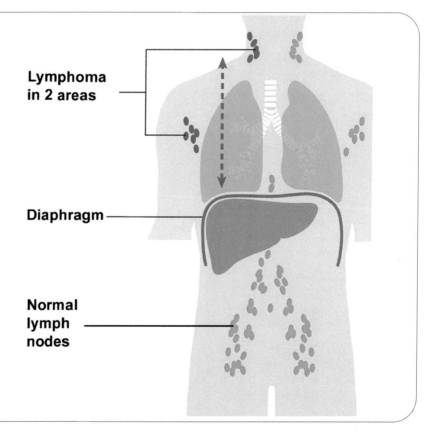

Lymphoma in 2 areas

Diaphragm

Normal lymph nodes

Stage 3

There is cancer in lymph tissue on both sides of the diaphragm.

Reproduced with permission by Cancer Research UK / Wikimedia Commons.

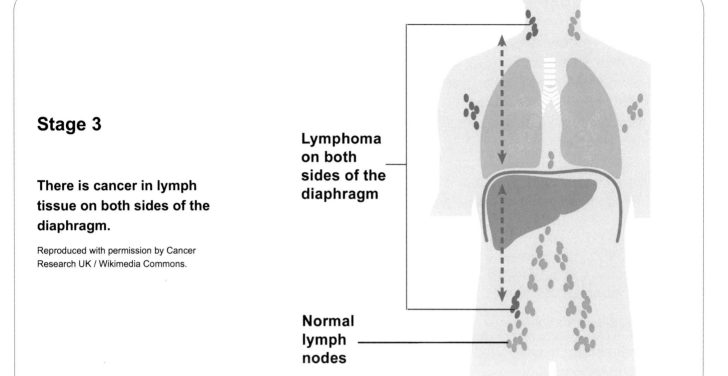

Lymphoma on both sides of the diaphragm

Normal lymph nodes

Stage 4

The cancer has widely spread outside the lymph system.

Reproduced with permission by Cancer Research UK / Wikimedia Commons

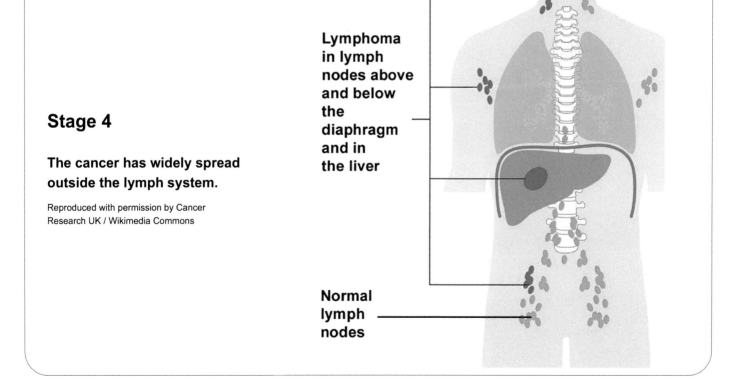

Lymphoma in lymph nodes above and below the diaphragm and in the liver

Normal lymph nodes

International Prognostic Index

The International Prognostic Index (IPI) is a scoring system for cancer prognosis. There is more than one version. The first IPI was created over 20 years ago. Other versions are adjusted for age or cancer stage. The NCCN-IPI is a newer version that works better than the first version.

Prognosis is based on risk factors. The risk factors included across IPI versions are alike.

> Older age

> High LDH level

> Poor performance status

> Advanced cancer stage

> Cancer spread outside lymph system (extranodal disease)

Points are assigned for each risk factor. There are four risk groups based on the total number of points.

> Low risk

> Low-intermediate risk

> High-intermediate risk

> High risk

CNS International Prognostic Index

The central nervous system (CNS) includes the brain and spinal cord. Although rare, DLBCL can spread to this system. To predict spread, doctors use the CNS International Prognostic Index. Six risk factors are used to score risk as low, intermediate, or high.

> Older age

> High LDH level

> Poor performance status

> Advanced cancer stage

> Extranodal disease in more than one body part

> Cancer spread to a kidney or adrenal gland

Biopsies

DLBCL can spread outside the lymph system. It is sometimes found in bone marrow at diagnosis. Rarely, it spreads into the CNS. A biopsy is needed to confirm cancer spread to these body parts.

Bone marrow biopsy

Tests on bone marrow are helpful for planning treatment. There are two methods of removing bone marrow.

> ➤ A bone marrow biopsy removes a core of bone and soft bone marrow.

> ➤ A bone marrow aspiration removes liquid bone marrow.

A bone marrow biopsy is not needed if cancer was detected in bone by PET/CT. If no cancer was detected in bone, a bone marrow biopsy is needed to confirm imaging results. Your doctor may want you to get an aspiration, too. Samples will be sent to a lab for cancer testing.

Lumbar puncture

Your doctor may suspect that the cancer has spread to your CNS. To confirm, a lumbar puncture (also called spinal tap) is needed. Spinal (or cerebrospinal) fluid will be removed. The sample will be sent to a lab for cancer testing.

Fertility and pregnancy care

Many younger people have healthy babies despite cancer and its treatment. If you wish to have a baby, there are important steps to take before treatment. Even if you are unsure, talk to your doctor.

Pregnancy test

Some cancer treatments can harm an unborn baby. Get a pregnancy test before treatment if you may be pregnant now. Your treatment options will depend on the results.

Birth control

During treatment, don't get pregnant or get someone pregnant. Take steps to prevent pregnancy. Your doctors can tell you which birth control methods are best to use.

Fertility counseling

Some cancer treatments can damage body parts that are needed to have a baby. Not being able to have a baby is called infertility. It can happen to people of any gender. Ask your cancer doctor if you are at risk for infertility.

You may receive a referral to a fertility specialist. A fertility specialist is an expert in helping people have babies. The fertility specialist can explain how you may be able to have a baby after treatment. Collecting and freezing sperm or eggs is a common method.

Review

- A complete report of your health is called a medical history. It includes any health problems you've had and diseases that run in your family.

- Tell your cancer doctors if you have recently had fevers, heavy sweats, or unexplained weight loss. These can be symptoms of lymphoma.

- A physical exam is a study of your body. Your cancer doctor will check if your lymph nodes, liver, or spleen are large.

- Performance status is a score of your ability to do day-to-day tasks. Doctors use it to assess if certain treatments are options.

- Your cancer doctors will decide if treatment is needed now using blood tests. They also use blood tests to look for signs of disease.

- Treatment for hepatitis and HIV is needed in order to safely receive strong cancer treatments.

- Imaging allows your doctors to see inside your body without cutting into it. It is used to assess what body parts may have cancer.

- You may undergo a heart test to see if it is safe to have certain cancer treatments.

- The cancer stage and prognostic scores are used to plan treatment.

- Lymphoma can spread to the middle of bone. A bone marrow biopsy with or without aspiration is needed for treatment planning.

- Lymphoma can spread to the central nervous system. Your doctor may order a lumbar puncture to test for cancer in this system.

- If you may be pregnant now, get a pregnancy test. Some cancer treatments can harm unborn babies.

- Ask your cancer doctors if you are at risk for infertility. There are ways to have a healthy baby after cancer treatment.

I am a giver and participant, however during treatment, it was time for me to receive. I had an AMAZING support team. My family, church, running club, golf group, book club, nurses, and doctors (oncologist, pulmonologist, cardiologist) all took GREAT care of me.

– Angie
   Survivor

4
Treatment options

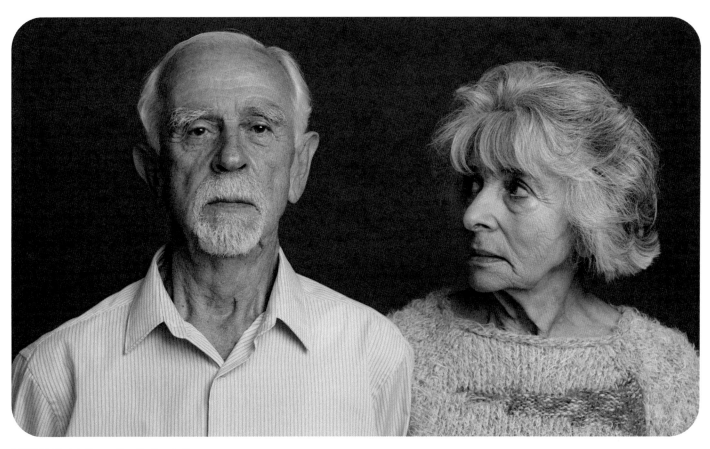

Treatment for DLBCL often has good results. Treatment options differ between people based on the cancer stage and other factors. Discuss with your doctors which options in this chapter are right for you.

Overview

Treatment for DLBCL includes treatment of the cancer and support for you. DLBCL is often cured. If a cure is not achieved, treatment can reduce symptoms, control cancer growth, and extend life. During and after cancer treatment, you may receive supportive care to improve your quality of life.

First-line treatment

First-line treatment is the first treatment or series of treatments received. Systemic therapy is very often the main treatment. It consists of medicines that travel through the bloodstream to treat cancer throughout the body.

A very common systemic therapy for DLBCL is chemoimmunotherapy. It consists of both chemotherapy and rituximab. It is given in cycles of treatment days followed by days of rest. This allows your body to recover before the next cycle.

Local treatment is also used as a first-line treatment. A local treatment targets cancer in a specific area. Involved-site radiation therapy (ISRT) is a local treatment for DLBCL. It is usually given in daily doses over several weeks.

Treatment response

Doctors assess treatment results with imaging. Positron emission tomography with diagnostic computed tomography (PET/CT) is used. Contrast is needed for the CT scan.

Scans done after treatment will be compared to scans before treatment. A biopsy may be needed to confirm imaging results. In the Lugano system, there are 4 types of responses:

> **Complete response** is the best result. Imaging detects less cancer to the extent that suggests a good outlook (prognosis). Organs are of normal size. Bone marrow is normal.

> **Partial response** is a decrease in cancer but less so than a complete response.

> **No response** is no clear change in the cancer. It is also called stable disease.

> **Progressive disease** is a worsening of the cancer.

Follow-up care

Follow-up care will be started if there's a complete response. Regular visits with your cancer doctor are needed. It is important to see a doctor who knows the health issues faced by lymphoma survivors. During follow-up care, you will be tested for cancer. Doctors call lymphoma that reappears on tests a relapse. Finding a relapse early will allow for timely treatment.

Second-line treatment

Second-line treatment is used for a cancer relapse. It is also used for cancers that didn't improve during first-line treatment. Doctors call these cancers refractory. Treatment options are based on whether a blood stem cell transplant is part of the treatment plan.

First-line treatment

Your doctors will plan your treatment based on many factors. A very important factor is the cancer stage. Treatment options by cancer stage are listed in Guide 3.

> Stage 1 and stage 2 cancers are treated alike because the extent of the cancer is limited.

> Stage 3 and stage 4 cancers are treated alike because the extent of the cancer is advanced.

Chemoimmunotherapy
Standard first-line treatment is RCHOP. RCHOP is often given in a 21-day cycle.

A 14-day cycle is noted as RCHOP-14. For some people, RCHOP may be too harmful, so a less harmful regimen may be used instead. For stages 1 and 2, treatment may consist of only ISRT if chemotherapy is not an option.

Stages 1 and 2
The outlook (prognosis) for stages 1 and 2 cancers is good. Treatment goals are to cure the cancer and limit toxic effects. To meet these goals, treatment options are based on the:

> size of the cancer; and

> International Prognostic Index (IPI) score.

Many people receive 6 cycles of RCHOP. If you won't receive radiation therapy, treatment

Guide 3
First-line treatment

Stage 1 **Stage 2**	When the cancer is small and the IPI score is 0, the 3 options are: • RCHOP-14 for 4 to 6 cycles • RCHOP-14 for 4 to 6 cycles followed by ISRT as listed in Guide 4 • RCHOP for 4 cycles followed by rituximab for 2 cycles
	When the cancer is small and the IPI score is 1 or higher, the 3 options are: • RCHOP for 3 cycles followed by ISRT as listed in Guide 4 • RCHOP for 6 cycles • RCHOP for 6 cycles followed by ISRT as listed in Guide 4
	When the cancer is large, the 2 options are: • RCHOP for 6 cycles • RCHOP for 6 cycles followed by ISRT as listed in Guide 4

Stage 3
Stage 4
	The 2 options are:
	• Clinical trial
	• RCHOP for 2 to 4 cycles then assess treatment results
	  • For a complete or partial response, complete 6 cycles of RCHOP
	  • For no response or progression, see Guide 6 and Guide 7 for options

results may be assessed after 3 to 4 cycles. Treatment plans may be changed based on results.

Fewer than 6 cycles may be an option if the outlook is very good. Cancers that are smaller than 7.5 cm (nonbulky) and an IPI score of 0 suggest excellent outcomes. Receiving fewer cycles reduces the toxic effects of treatment.

When all cycles of RCHOP are finished, treatment results will be assessed. If your treatment plan includes ISRT, read the section called *ISRT* on the next page. If ISRT wasn't planned, the next steps of treatment are:

> Start follow-up care if a complete response has been achieved.

> Start second-line treatment if there was less than a complete response. A second option for a partial response is ISRT.

Stages 3 and 4

At the time of diagnosis, DLBCL is stage 3 or 4 in more than half of people. Treatment can provide long-term control for many people.

A clinical trial may be an option. Ask your treatment team if there is a clinical trial that is right for you. Clinical trials can answer questions, such as:

> Is radiation therapy to large (bulky) areas of advanced cancer helpful?

> Is radiation therapy to areas other than lymph nodes helpful for advanced cancer?

> Does lenalidomide or an autologous transplant after RCHOP help stop relapse? Who benefits from this treatment?

Systemic therapy
First-line regimens

Preferred regimens
· RCHOP (21- or 14-day cycle)

Other regimens
Fit adults
· Dose-adjusted EPOCH and rituximab
Adults with heart problems
· RCEPP
· RCDOP
· Dose-adjusted EPOCH and rituximab
· RCEOP
· RGCVP
Frail adults or older, sick adults
· RCEPP
· RCDOP
· R-mini-CHOP
· RGCVP

Acronyms

EPOCH = etoposide, prednisone, vincristine, cyclophosphamide, doxorubicin

RCDOP = rituximab, cyclophosphamide, liposomal doxorubicin, vincristine, prednisone

RCEOP = rituximab, cyclophosphamide, etoposide, vincristine, prednisone

RCEPP = rituximab, cyclophosphamide, etoposide, prednisone, procarbazine

RCHOP = rituximab, cyclophosphamide, doxorubicin, vincristine, prednisone

RGCVP = rituximab, gemcitabine, cyclophosphamide, vincristine, prednisolone

For advanced cancer, standard treatment is 6 cycles of RCHOP. Treatment results will be assessed after 2 to 4 cycles. If there was a partial or complete response, complete the 6 cycles of RCHOP. If RCHOP didn't work, read *Second-line treatment* for options.

Treatment results will be assessed again after the 6 cycles are completed. After a complete response, ISRT is an option if there was bulky areas or cancer in bone. If there was less than a complete response, read *Second-line treatment* for options.

Sometimes DLBCL spreads into the central nervous system (CNS). This system includes your brain and spinal cord. Most CNS disease can be treated with methotrexate.

ISRT
For stages 1 and 2, ISRT after RCHOP may help cure the cancer in more people. It is not given to all limited cancers but to cancers more likely to relapse. For testicular lymphoma, scrotal radiation therapy is used instead of ISRT.

When all the cycles of RCHOP are finished, treatment results will be assessed. For PET/CT, radiologists use the PET Five-Point Scale (5-PS) to report results. ISRT options by treatment response are listed in Guide 4.

For a complete response, ISRT as planned is an option. For a partial response, the options are higher-dose ISRT, autologous transplant, and a clinical trial based on 5-PS scores. If there was no response or progression, read *Second-line treatment* for options.

When ISRT is finished, treatment results will be checked again. It may take weeks for the true results to be seen. PET/CT should occur at least 8 weeks after treatment.

Guide 4
ISRT for stages 1 and 2

Complete response to RCHOP	ISRT with standard radiation dose
Partial response to RCHOP	For a PET Five-Point Scale of 4, the option is: • ISRT with higher radiation dose For a PET Five-Point Scale of 5, the 3 options are: • ISRT with higher radiation dose • Autologous transplant with or without ISRT if 6 cycles of RCHOP or 4 to 6 cycles of RCHOP-14 were completed • Clinical trial
No response or progression	See Guide 6 and Guide 7 for treatment options

Follow-up care

Follow-up care is important for your long-term health. It is started when a complete response has been achieved. Your cancer doctor will provide you with a follow-up care plan.

While DLBCL can be cured, it is very important to monitor for the return of the cancer. The return of cancer is called a relapse. Tests for a relapse include medical history, physical exam, and blood tests. Some people also get imaging. The schedule for these tests is listed in Guide 5.

Guide 5 Follow-up care	
	Get these tests:
Medical history, Physical exam, and blood tests	• Every 3 to 6 months for 5 years after treatment • Every year starting in the sixth year after treatment • As needed
CT scan with contrast of the chest, abdomen, and pelvis or PET/CT if cancer is only detected with this method	For stage 1 and 2, get imaging as needed
	For stage 3 and 4, get imaging: • Not more often than every 6 months for 2 years after treatment • As needed

Second-line treatment

Sometimes chemoimmunotherapy works but the cancer returns. Sometimes, chemoimmunotherapy doesn't work enough or at all. In these cases, second-line treatments are used.

Your treatment options will depend on if you can have a blood stem cell transplant. Doctors decide whether a transplant is an option based on many factors, such as:

> Illnesses other than cancer

> How well organs are working

> What you want

Stem cell transplant

If a transplant is planned, the first step of care is to receive systemic therapy. Second-line regimens consist of chemotherapy. Rituximab may be added.

Systemic therapy is given to reduce the amount of cancer in your body. It is also given to assess how well a transplant will work. Transplants are more successful when systemic therapy has good results. See Guide 6 for a list of options based on results of the systemic therapy.

After systemic therapy, a clinical trial may be an option. There may be a clinical trial on transplants or a new treatment.

For a complete or partial response, an autologous transplant is commonly done. For a select group of people, an allogeneic transplant is an option. After either transplant, ISRT may be added to treat a certain area.

For less than a complete response, anti-CD19 CAR T-cell therapy may be an option. This type of treatment includes axicabtagene ciloleucel and tisagenlecleucel. To receive either treatment, you must have received two or more chemoimmunotherapy regimens in the past. You must not have received CAR T-cell therapy in the past.

For no response or progression, other options are systemic therapy and supportive care. A different second-line regimen may work better than the one you had. Supportive care includes treatment for health issues caused by cancer or its treatment. ISRT may reduce discomfort caused by the cancer.

Guide 6
Stem cell transplant

The first step of care is to receive systemic therapy and assess the results:

Complete response	The 5 options are: • Autologous transplant • Autologous transplant followed by ISRT • Clinical trial • Allogeneic transplant in certain cases • Allogeneic transplant in certain cases followed by ISRT
Partial response	The 6 options are: • Anti-CD19 CAR T-cell therapy • Autologous transplant • Autologous transplant followed by ISRT • Clinical trial • Allogeneic transplant in certain cases • Allogeneic transplant in certain cases followed by ISRT
No response or progression	The 4 options are: • Anti-CD19 CAR T-cell therapy • Clinical trial • Second- and third-line systemic therapy • Supportive care including ISRT

Other second-line treatments

There are treatment options other than transplants that may relieve symptoms and prolong life. If a transplant is not planned, see Guide 7 for treatment options.

A clinical trial may be an option. Ask your treatment team if there's one that is right for you. Also, a systemic therapy may slow the growth of the cancer.

If the cancer relapses or is refractory more than once, anti-CD19 CAR T-cell therapy may be an option. This treatment includes axicabtagene ciloleucel and tisagenlecleucel. To receive either treatment, you must have received two or more chemoimmunotherapy regimens in the past. You must not have received CAR T-cell therapy in the past.

Symptoms caused by the cancer or its treatment may be relieved with supportive care. Supportive care aims to improve quality of life. For example, ISRT may reduce discomfort caused by the cancer.

Guide 7
Second-line treatment if transplant not planned

One relapse or refractory cancer	The 3 options are: • Clinical trial • Second-line systemic therapy • Supportive care including ISRT
Two or more relapses or refractory cancer	The 4 options are: • Anti-CD19 CAR T-cell therapy • Clinical trial • Second- and third-line systemic therapy • Supportive care including ISRT

Systemic therapy
Second- and third-line regimens

Regimens for when a transplant is part of treatment plan

Preferred regimens
- DHAP with or without rituximab
- DHAX with or without rituximab
- GDP with or without rituximab
- ICE with or without rituximab

Other regimens
- ESHAP with or without rituximab
- GemOx with or without rituximab
- MINE with or without rituximab

Regimens for when a transplant is not part of treatment plan

Preferred regimens
- GemOX with or without rituximab
- Polatuzumab vedotin with or without rituximab and with or without bendamustine

Other regimens
- CEPP with or without rituximab
- CEOP with or without rituximab
- Dose-adjusted EPOCH with or without rituximab

Other regimens continued
- GDP with or without rituximab
- Gemcitabine and vinorelbine with or without rituximab
- Rituximab
- Tafasitamab-cxix and lenalidomide

Useful in some cases
- Brentuximab vedotin for CD30-positive DLBCL
- Bendamustine with or without rituximab
- Ibrutinib for non-GCB DLBCL
- Lenalidomide with or without rituximab for non-GCB DLBCL

Anti-CD19 CAR T-cell therapy
- Axicabtagene ciloleucel
- Tisagenlecleucel

Third-line regimen including after a transplant or CAR T-cell therapy
- Selinexor

Acronyms

CEPP = cyclophosphamide, etoposide, prednisone, procarbazine

CEOP = cyclophosphamide, etoposide, vincristine, prednisone

DHAP = dexamethasone, cisplatin, cytarabine

DHAX = dexamethasone, cytarabine, oxaliplatin

GDP = gemcitabine, dexamethasone, (cisplatin or carboplatin)

ICE = ifosfamide, carboplatin, etoposide

EPOCH = etoposide, prednisone, vincristine, cyclophosphamide, doxorubicin

ESHAP = etoposide, methylprednisolone, cytarabine, cisplatin

GemOx = gemcitabine, oxaliplatin

Supportive care

Supportive care aims to improve your quality of life. It is sometimes called palliative care. It's important for everyone, not just people at the end of life. Talk with your treatment team to plan the best supportive care for you.

Supportive care can address many needs. It can prevent or relieve emotional or physical symptoms. It can also help with making treatment decisions. Supportive care also includes help with coordination of care between health providers.

Treatment side effects

All cancer treatments can cause unwanted health issues. Such health issues are called side effects. Some side effects may be harmful to your health. Others may just be unpleasant.

Side effects differ between people. Some people have side effects while others have none. Some people have mild side effects while others have severe effects. Side effects depend on the treatment type, length or dose of treatment, and the person.

Most side effects appear shortly after treatment starts and will stop after treatment. However, other side effects are long-term or may appear years later. Ask your treatment team for a complete list of side effects of your treatments.

Tell your treatment team about any new or worse symptoms you get. There may be ways to help you feel better. There are also ways to prevent some side effects.

Read more about side effects of CAR T-cell therapy in *NCCN Guidelines for Patients: Immunotherapy Side Effects*, availalble at NCCN.org/patientguidelines.

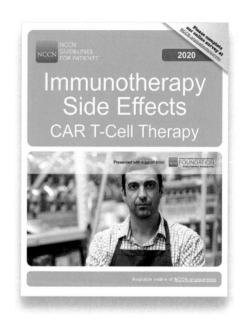

Review

> DLBCL is often cured. If a cure is not achieved, treatment can reduce symptoms, control cancer growth, and extend life.

> First-line treatment often consists of a chemoimmunotherapy called RCHOP. ISRT may be given after RCHOP to help stop the cancer from coming back.

> PET/CT scans are used to assess the results of treatment. There are four groups of treatment response. From best to worst, they are called a complete response, partial response, no response, and progressive disease.

> Follow-up care is started when a complete response has been achieved. It includes regular visits with a cancer doctor and testing for cancer.

> Second-line treatment is based on whether a blood stem cell transplant is planned. Autologous transplant is more commonly done than allogeneic transplants. Besides transplants, the options are chemotherapy with or without rituxumab, anti-CD19 CAR T-cell therapy, clinical trials, and supportive care.

> Besides cancer treatment, you may receive supportive care to prevent or reduce symptoms related to the cancer or its treatment.

5
Making treatment decisions

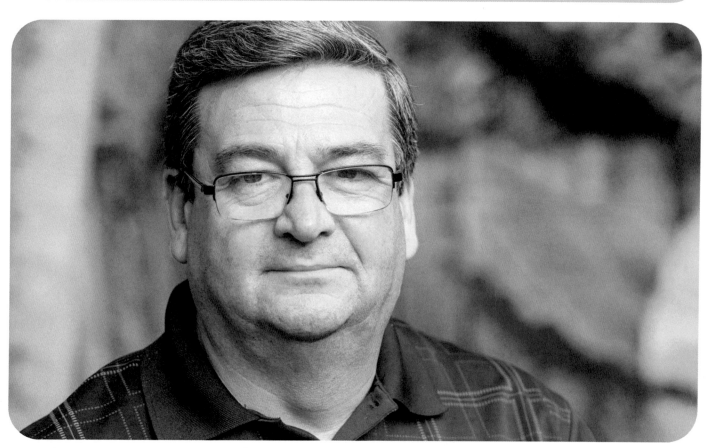

It's important to be comfortable with the cancer treatment you choose. This choice starts with having an open and honest conversation with your doctors.

It's your choice

In shared decision-making, you and your doctors share information, discuss the options, and agree on a treatment plan. It starts with an open and honest conversation between you and your doctor.

Treatment decisions are very personal. What is important to you may not be important to someone else.

Some things that may play a role in your decisions:

> What you want and how that might differ from what others want

> Your religious and spiritual beliefs

> Your feelings about certain treatments like surgery or chemotherapy

> Your feelings about pain or side effects such as nausea and vomiting

> Cost of treatment, travel to treatment centers, and time away from work

> Quality of life and length of life

> How active you are and the activities that are important to you

Think about what you want from treatment. Discuss openly the risks and benefits of specific treatments and procedures. Weigh options and share concerns with your doctor. If you take the time to build a relationship with your doctor, it

will help you feel supported when considering options and making treatment decisions.

Second opinion

It is normal to want to start treatment as soon as possible. While cancer can't be ignored, there is time to have another doctor review your test results and suggest a treatment plan. This is called getting a second opinion, and it's a normal part of cancer care. Even doctors get second opinions!

Things you can do to prepare:

> Check with your insurance company about its rules on second opinions. There may be out-of-pocket costs to see doctors who are not part of your insurance plan.

> Make plans to have copies of all your records sent to the doctor you will see for your second opinion.

Support groups

Many people diagnosed with cancer find support groups to be helpful. Support groups often include people at different stages of treatment. Some people may be newly diagnosed, while others may be finished with treatment. If your hospital or community doesn't have support groups for people with cancer, check out the websites listed in this book.

Questions to ask your doctors

Possible questions to ask your doctors are listed on the following pages. Feel free to use these questions or come up with your own. Be clear about your goals for treatment and find out what to expect from treatment.

Questions to ask about testing and staging

1. What tests will I have?

2. When will I have a biopsy? Will I have more than one? What are the risks? Is it painful?

3. How do I prepare for testing?

4. What if I am pregnant?

5. Where do I go to get tested? How long will the tests take and will any test hurt?

6. Should I bring someone with me? Should I bring a list of my medications?

7. How soon will I know the results and who will explain them to me?

8. Would you give me a copy of the pathology report and other test results?

9. What type of lymphoma do I have? Where did it start in my body?

10. What is the cancer stage? Does this stage mean the cancer has spread far?

11. Is this a fast- or slow-growing cancer?

12. Can this cancer be cured? If not, how well can treatment stop the cancer from growing?

13. Who will talk with me about the next steps? When?

Questions to ask about treatment options

1. What are my treatment options? Are you suggesting options other than what NCCN recommends? If yes, why?

2. Do your suggested options include clinical trials? Please explain why.

3. What will happen if I do nothing?

4. How do my age, overall health, and other factors affect my options? What if I am pregnant or planning to get pregnant?

5. Does any option offer a cure or long-term cancer control? Are my chances any better for one option than another? Less time-consuming? Less expensive?

6. How do you know if treatment is working? How will I know if treatment is working?

7. What are my options if treatment stops working?

8. What are the possible complications? What are the short- and long-term side effects of treatment?

9. How will treatment affect my looks, speech, chewing, and swallowing? Will my sense of smell or taste change?

10. What can be done to prevent or relieve the side effects of treatment?

11. What supportive care services are available to me during and after treatment?

12. Can I stop treatment at any time? What will happen if I stop treatment?

Questions to ask about clinical trials

1. Are there clinical trials for my type of cancer?

2. What are the treatments used in the clinical trial?

3. What does the treatment do?

4. Has the treatment been used before? Has it been used for other types of cancer?

5. What are the risks and benefits of joining the clinical trial and the treatment being tested?

6. What side effects should I expect? How will the side effects be controlled?

7. How long will I be in the clinical trial?

8. Will I be able to get other treatment if this doesn't work?

9. How will you know the treatment is working?

10. Will the clinical trial cost me anything? If so, how much?

Questions to ask about getting treatment

1. Will I have to go to the hospital or elsewhere? How often? How long is each visit?

2. What do I need to think about if I will travel for treatment?

3. Do I have a choice of when to begin treatment? Can I choose the days and times of treatment?

4. How do I prepare for treatment? Do I have to stop taking any of my medicines? Are there foods I will have to avoid?

5. Should I bring someone with me when I get treated?

6. Will the treatment hurt?

7. How much will the treatment cost me? What does my insurance cover?

8. Will I miss work or school? Will I be able to drive?

9. Is home care after treatment needed? If yes, what type?

10. How soon will I be able to manage my own health?

11. When will I be able to return to my normal activities?

Websites

American Cancer Society
cancer.org/cancer/non-hodgkin-lymphoma

Leukemia & Lymphoma Society
LLS.org/informationspecialists

National Cancer Institute (NCI)
cancer.gov/types/lymphoma

National Coalition for Cancer Survivorship
canceradvocacy.org/toolbox

NCCN Patient Resources
NCCN.org/patients

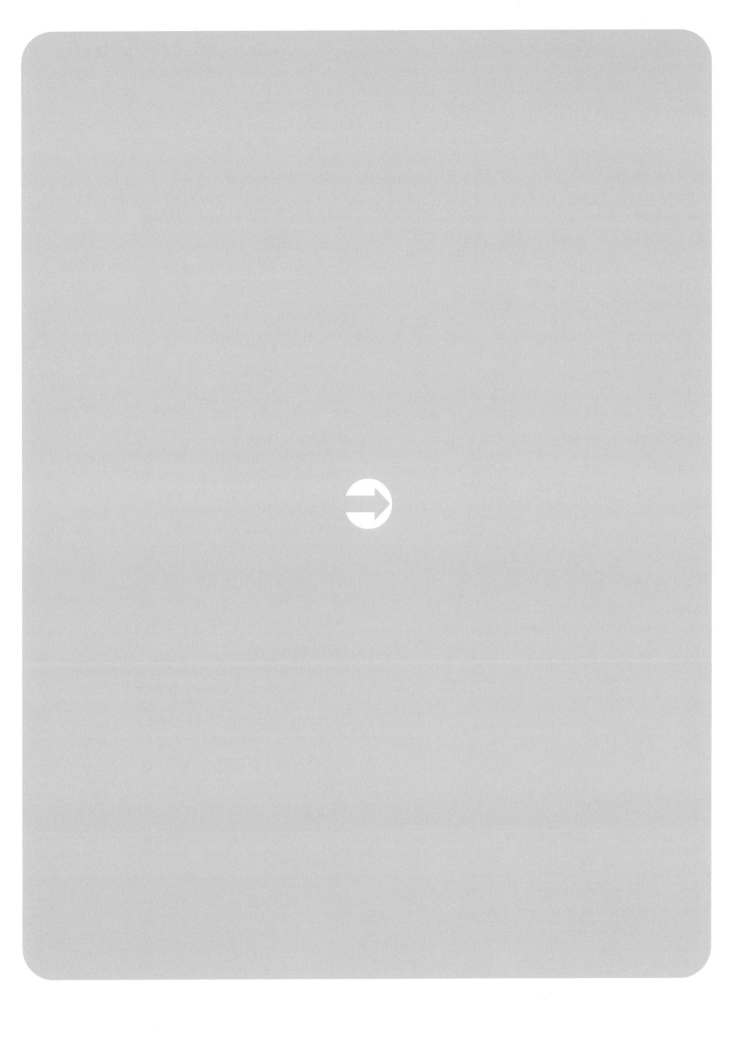

Words to know

adrenal gland
A small organ on top of each kidney that makes hormones.

allogeneic stem cell transplant
A cancer treatment that replaces abnormal blood stem cells with healthy donor cells. Also called allogeneic hematopoietic cell transplant.

autologous blood stem cell transplant
A cancer treatment that destroys cancer cells with intense treatment then rebuilds destroyed bone marrow with your own healthy blood stem cells. Also called an HDT/ASCR (high-dose therapy with autologous stem cell rescue).

B cell
A type of a white blood cell called a lymphocyte. Also called B lymphocyte.

B symptoms
Fevers, heavy sweats, and unexpected weight loss caused by B-cell cancers.

beta-2 microglobulin
A small protein made by many types of cells.

biopsy
A procedure that removes fluid or tissue samples to be tested for a disease.

bone marrow
The sponge-like tissue in the center of most bones.

bone marrow aspiration
A procedure that removes a liquid bone marrow sample to test for a disease.

bone marrow biopsy
A procedure that removes bone and solid bone marrow samples to test for a disease.

cancer stage
A rating of the outlook of a cancer based on its growth and spread.

chemotherapy
Cancer drugs that stop the cell life cycle so cells don't increase in number.

clinical trial
A type of research that assesses how well health tests or treatments work in people.

CNS
central nervous system

complete blood count (CBC)
A lab test that measures the number of red blood cells, white blood cells, and platelets.

complete response
An absence of all signs and symptoms of cancer after treatment.

computed tomography (CT)
A test that uses x-rays from many angles to make a picture of the insides of the body.

contrast
A substance put into your body to make clearer pictures during imaging tests.

corticosteroid
A drug used to reduce redness, swelling, and pain, but also to kill cancer cells.

deoxyribonucleic acid (DNA)
A chain of chemicals in cells that contains coded instructions for making and controlling cells.

diagnosis
An identification of an illness based on tests.

diaphragm
A sheet of muscles below the ribs that helps a person to breathe.

differential
A lab test of the number of white blood cells for each type.

DLBCL
diffuse large B-cell lymphoma

echocardiogram
A test that uses sound waves to make pictures of the heart.

endoscopy
A procedure to work inside the digestive tract with a device that is guided through natural openings.

fertility specialist
An expert who helps people to have babies.

flow cytometry
A lab test of substances on the surface of cells to identify the type of cells present.

fluorescence in situ hybridization (FISH)
A lab test that uses special dyes to look for abnormal chromosomes and genes.

FNA
fine-needle aspiration

gene
Coded instructions in cells for making new cells and controlling how cells behave.

germinal center
A short-lived structure that forms within an lymphatic organ in response to germs.

GCB
germinal center B-cell

HDT-ASCR
high-dose therapy-autologous stem cell rescue

imaging
A test that makes pictures (images) of the insides of the body.

immune system
The body's natural defense against disease.

immunohistochemistry (IHC)
A lab test of cancer cells to find specific cell traits involved in abnormal cell growth.

immunomodulator
A cancer drug that modifies some parts of the body's disease-fighting system.

International Prognostic Index (IPI)
A scoring system used to predict the outcome of diffuse large B-cell lymphoma.

involved-site radiation therapy (ISRT)
Treatment with radiation that is delivered to areas with cancer growth at diagnosis.

karyotype
A lab test that makes a map of chromosomes to find defects.

kidney
One of a pair of organs that removes waste from blood, helps control blood pressure, and helps to make red blood cells.

kinase inhibitor
A drug that blocks the transfer of phosphate.

lactate dehydrogenase (LDH)
A protein that helps to make energy in cells.

lumbar puncture
A procedure that removes spinal fluid with a needle. Also called a spinal tap.

lymph
A clear fluid containing white blood cells.

lymph node
A small, bean-shaped, disease-fighting structure.

lymph system
A network of organs and vessels that collects and transports a fluid called lymph.

lymphocyte
One of three main types of white blood cells that help protect the body from illness.

lymphoma
A cancer of white blood cells called lymphocytes that are within the lymph system.

magnetic resonance imaging (MRI)
A test that uses a magnetic field and radio waves to make pictures of the insides of the body.

medical history
A report of all your health events and medications.

monoclonal antibody
A type of cancer drug that stops growth signals.

multigated acquisition (MUGA) scan
A test that uses radiation to make pictures of the heart.

physical exam
A study of the body by a health expert for signs of disease.

positron emission tomography (PET)
A test that uses radioactive material to see the shape and function of body parts.

prognosis
The likely course and outcome of a disease based on tests.

radiation therapy
A treatment that uses intense energy to kill cancer cells.

relapse
The return of cancer after a period of improvement.

side effect
An unhealthy or unpleasant physical or emotional response to treatment.

spleen
An organ to the left of the stomach that helps protect the body from disease.

supportive care
Health care that includes symptom relief but not cancer treatment. Also called palliative care.

T cell
A type of a white blood cell called a lymphocyte.

TLS
tumor lysis syndrome

uric acid
A chemical that is made and released into the blood when cells and other substances in the body break down.

white blood cell
A type of blood cell that fights disease and infection.

NCCN Contributors

This patient guide is based on the NCCN Clinical Practice Guidelines in Oncology (NCCN Guidelines®) for B-Cell Lymphomas. It was adapted, reviewed, and published with help from the following people:

Dorothy A. Shead, MS
Director, Patient Information Operations

Laura J. Hanisch, PsyD
Medical Writer/Patient Information Specialist

Erin Vidic, MA
Medical Writer

Rachael Clarke
Senior Medical Copyeditor

Tanya Fischer, MEd, MSLIS
Medical Writer

Kim Williams
Creative Services Manager

Susan Kidney
Design Specialist

The NCCN Guidelines® for B-Cell Lymphomas, Version 4.2020 were developed by the following NCCN Panel Members:

Andrew D. Zelenetz, MD, PhD/Chair
Memorial Sloan Kettering Cancer Center

Leo I. Gordon, MD/Co-Vice Chair
Robert H. Lurie Comprehensive Cancer Center of Northwestern University

Jeremy S. Abramson, MD
Massachusetts General Hospital Cancer Center

Ranjana H. Advani, MD
Stanford Cancer Institute

Nancy L. Bartlett, MD
Siteman Cancer Center at Barnes-Jewish Hospital and Washington University School of Medicine

L. Elizabeth Budde, MD, PhD
City of Hope National Medical Center

Paolo F. Caimi, MD
Case Comprehensive Cancer Center/ University Hospitals Seidman Cancer Center and Cleveland Clinic Taussig Cancer Institute

Julie E. Chang, MD
University of Wisconsin Carbone Cancer Center

Julio C. Chavez, MD
Moffitt Cancer Center

* **Beth Christian, MD**
James Cancer Hospital and Solove Research Institute

Sven De Vos, MD, PhD
UCLA Jonsson Comprehensive Cancer Center

Bita Fakhri, MD
UCSF Helen Diller Family Comprehensive Cancer Center

Luis E. Fasyad, MD
The University of Texas MD Anderson Cancer Center

Martha J. Glenn, MD
Huntsman Cancer Institute at the University of Utah

Thomas M. Habermann, MD
Mayo Clinic Cancer Center

Francisco Hernandez-Ilizaliturri, MD
Roswell Park Cancer Institute

Mark S. Kaminski, MD
University of Michigan Rogel Cancer Center

Christopher R. Kelsey, MD
Duke Cancer Institute

Nadia Khan, MD
Fox Chase Cancer Center

* **Susan Krivacic, MPAff**
Consultant

Ann S. LaCasce, MD
Dana-Farber/Brigham and Women's Cancer Center

Amitkumar Mehta MD
O'Neal Comprehensive Cancer Center at UAB

Auayporn Nademanee, MD
City of Hope National Medical Center

Mayur Narkhede, MD
O'Neal Comprehensive Cancer Center at UAB

* **Rachel Rabinovitch, MD**
University of Colorado Cancer Center

Nishitha Reddy, MD
Vanderbilt-Ingram Cancer Center

Erin Reid, MD
UC San Diego Moores Cancer Center

Kenneth B. Roberts, MD
Yale Cancer Center/Smilow Cancer Hospital

Stephen D. Smith, MD
Fred Hutchinson Cancer Research Center/ Seattle Cancer Care Alliance

Jakub Svoboda, MD
Abramson Cancer Center at the University of Pennsylvania

Lode J. Swinnen, MB, ChB
The Sidney Kimmel Comprehensive Cancer Center at Johns Hopkins

Julie M. Vose, MD, MBA
Fred & Pamela Buffett Cancer Center

NCCN Staff

Mary Dwyer, MS
Director, Guidelines Operations

Hema Sundar, PhD
Oncology Scientist/Senior Medical Writer

* Reviewed this patient guide. For disclosures, visit NCCN.org/about/disclosure.aspx.

NCCN Cancer Centers

Abramson Cancer Center
at the University of Pennsylvania
Philadelphia, Pennsylvania
800.789.7366 • pennmedicine.org/cancer

Fred & Pamela Buffett Cancer Center
Omaha, Nebraska
800.999.5465 • nebraskamed.com/cancer

Case Comprehensive Cancer Center/
University Hospitals Seidman Cancer
Center and Cleveland Clinic Taussig
Cancer Institute
Cleveland, Ohio
800.641.2422 • UH Seidman Cancer Center
uhhospitals.org/services/cancer-services
866.223.8100 • CC Taussig Cancer Institute
my.clevelandclinic.org/departments/cancer
216.844.8797 • Case CCC
case.edu/cancer

City of Hope National Medical Center
Los Angeles, California
800.826.4673 • cityofhope.org

Dana-Farber/Brigham and
Women's Cancer Center
Massachusetts General Hospital
Cancer Center
Boston, Massachusetts
877.332.4294
dfbwcc.org
massgeneral.org/cancer

Duke Cancer Institute
Durham, North Carolina
888.275.3853 • dukecancerinstitute.org

Fox Chase Cancer Center
Philadelphia, Pennsylvania
888.369.2427 • foxchase.org

Huntsman Cancer Institute
at the University of Utah
Salt Lake City, Utah
877.585.0303
huntsmancancer.org

Fred Hutchinson Cancer
Research Center/Seattle
Cancer Care Alliance
Seattle, Washington
206.288.7222 • seattlecca.org
206.667.5000 • fredhutch.org

The Sidney Kimmel Comprehensive
Cancer Center at Johns Hopkins
Baltimore, Maryland
410.955.8964
hopkinsmedicine.org/kimmel_cancer_center

Robert H. Lurie Comprehensive
Cancer Center of Northwestern
University
Chicago, Illinois
866.587.4322 • cancer.northwestern.edu

Mayo Clinic Cancer Center
Phoenix/Scottsdale, Arizona
Jacksonville, Florida
Rochester, Minnesota
800.446.2279 • Arizona
904.953.0853 • Florida
507.538.3270 • Minnesota
mayoclinic.org/departments-centers/mayo-clinic-cancer-center

Memorial Sloan Kettering
Cancer Center
New York, New York
800.525.2225 • mskcc.org

Moffitt Cancer Center
Tampa, Florida
800.456.3434 • moffitt.org

The Ohio State University
Comprehensive Cancer Center -
James Cancer Hospital and
Solove Research Institute
Columbus, Ohio
800.293.5066 • cancer.osu.edu

O'Neal Comprehensive
Cancer Center at UAB
Birmingham, Alabama
800.822.0933 • uab.edu/onealcancercenter

Roswell Park Comprehensive
Cancer Center
Buffalo, New York
877.275.7724 • roswellpark.org

Siteman Cancer Center at Barnes-
Jewish Hospital and Washington
University School of Medicine
St. Louis, Missouri
800.600.3606 • siteman.wustl.edu

St. Jude Children's Research Hospital
The University of Tennessee
Health Science Center
Memphis, Tennessee
888.226.4343 • stjude.org
901.683.0055 • westclinic.com

Stanford Cancer Institute
Stanford, California
877.668.7535 • cancer.stanford.edu

UC San Diego Moores Cancer Center
La Jolla, California
858.657.7000 • cancer.ucsd.edu

UCLA Jonsson
Comprehensive Cancer Center
Los Angeles, California
310.825.5268 • cancer.ucla.edu

UCSF Helen Diller Family
Comprehensive Cancer Center
San Francisco, California
800.689.8273 • cancer.ucsf.edu

University of Colorado Cancer Center
Aurora, Colorado
720.848.0300 • coloradocancercenter.org

University of Michigan
Rogel Cancer Center
Ann Arbor, Michigan
800.865.1125 • rogelcancercenter.org

The University of Texas
MD Anderson Cancer Center
Houston, Texas
800.392.1611 • mdanderson.org

University of Wisconsin
Carbone Cancer Center
Madison, Wisconsin
608.265.1700 • uwhealth.org/cancer

UT Southwestern Simmons
Comprehensive Cancer Center
Dallas, Texas
214.648.3111 • utswmed.org/cancer

Vanderbilt-Ingram Cancer Center
Nashville, Tennessee
800.811.8480 • vicc.org

Yale Cancer Center/
Smilow Cancer Hospital
New Haven, Connecticut
855.4.SMILOW • yalecancercenter.org

Notes

Index